Put Your Mask on First!

The Caregiver's Guide to Self-Care

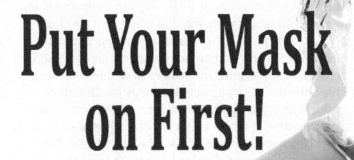

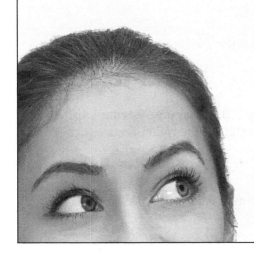

Dr. Gary Bradt
Scott Silknitter

Disclaimer

This book is for informational purposes only and is not intended as medical advice, diagnosis, or treatment. Always seek advice from a qualified physician about medical concerns, and do not disregard medical advice because of something you may read within this book. This book does not replace the needs for diagnostic evaluation, ongoing physician care, and professional assessment of treatments. Every effort has been made to make this book as complete and helpful as possible. It is important, however, for this book to be used as a resource and idea-generating guide and not as an ultimate source for plan of care.

ISBN 978-1-943285-90-7

Published by
R.O.S. Therapy Systems, L.L.C.
Greensboro, NC
888-352-9788
www.ROSTherapySystems.com

Table of Contents

Family Members and Caregivers that have read this book:

_____

_____

_____

_____

_____

_____

_____

_____

_____

_____

_____

_____

_____

_____

Introduction

You are a caregiver—your loved one may have one or more of the following ailments: Heart Disease, Alzheimer's, Parkinson's, Frontal Lobe Dementia, Diabetes, had a Stroke or has a Visual Impairment, or has some combination of various issues.

No matter what the issue is, we know for sure that your loved one did not choose to get it, and you did not choose to be a caregiver, but both things have happened.

You can remember the day your loved one received a life-changing diagnosis like it was yesterday.

- Roger, you have Parkinson's disease.

- Mary, you have Alzheimer's.

- Susan had a stroke.

- Scott, you have cancer.

- There has been an accident, and Steven suffered a brain injury.

You will never forget the moment that changed your lives forever. For some, it was an immediate shock with no time for planning or research. For others, it was a slow progression that started with searching for an answer or a cure, while all the worrying about symptoms and possibilities began to wear you out.

Consider the couple from Texas that spent a year with various specialists trying to figure out why a 45-year-old father of four had a tremor in his right hand. It was first noticed at a surprise wedding anniversary party that their kids had planned. After a year of tests, he was told that he had Parkinson's. He was also told that he should expect to lose control of his bodily functions, that he will need a walker, that he will become bedridden, and he will die because the medicine will only work for so long.

There is also the 60-year-old who just retired after 35 years as a teacher. She and her husband were going to begin traveling the world and spending time with children and grandchildren when a phone call came. Her mother, with Alzheimer's, was going to have to live with them, and the daughter would be her caregiver. As weeks turned into months and months turned into years, resentment and anger built up inside the daughter.

Things were not supposed to be this way. She was supposed to be traveling and enjoying retirement, not stuck in her house caring for her mother who did not recognize her most of the time, and was becoming quite mean as well.

A vicious cycle was forming: first, feeling angry toward her mother and then, feeling guilty for feeling angry. She knew it was not her mother's fault for being sick, and there was nowhere else for her mother to go. Nevertheless, all of the stress was beginning to wear the daughter out.

The stories may be different, but the results are the same: None of us that are caregivers expected it to happen, but one day we received the news that changed our lives.

Fast forward a few months, or even years, from that day, and we are now full-time caregivers. Does any of this feel or sound familiar?

You're tired.

That is an understatement. You are exhausted. The 24/7 job is taking its toll. Every few months, your loved one's sleep patterns go out of whack. This always seems to happen with medication changes or when family comes to visit.

You worry about money.

This is a constant struggle.

Scenario 1: You worked hard your whole life. You played by the rules. You have the pension money and Social Security coming in, but it seems like there is less and less each month as you need different items that aren't covered by insurance or Medicare.

Scenario 2: You work a full-time job and are trying to raise your kids and take care of your mom, who is now living with you. As the kids get older, their needs get more and more expensive. As your mom's health issue progresses, it seems her needs become more and more expensive and for some reason, Medicare does not seem to cover the little day-to-day things that she really needs. You are beginning to feel strapped.

<u>You feel alone and isolated.</u>

Every day you get up and go through your routine. As your loved one's issues progress, and they have issues with eating, talking, using the bathroom, or just walking, you spend more time in the house. When you do get out, it is just to run an errand as quickly as possible, so you can get your loved one back home. Most of your friends stop calling or coming

by because they have their own issues.
Your kids have their own lives
and families, and you realize that former
co-workers really were just that—
co-workers—not friends.

<u>You're sad about the things that you were supposed to do together and now know you never will.</u>

Scenario 1: This was supposed to be
the time that you were going to sleep in,
travel, go out for nights on the town,
and basically do whatever you wanted
to do, whenever you wanted to do it.
But a medical malady has struck and
being a full-time caregiver is now
your lot.

Scenario 2: Your kids are finally old
enough to be self-sufficient. You do not
have to take them everywhere all of the
time. But, instead of being able to go out to
dinner more and enjoy "date nights" with
your special someone, you are now
spending each night at home taking care of

them instead, due to an unforeseen medical malady that has befallen them.

You get mad at your loved one and then feel guilty because you know they did not choose to be here.

It did not start out this way, but lately, when you hear your loved one calling for you, you begin to cringe when you hear their voice. You are tired of being alone, and you start to blame them because their disease is cheating you of what was supposed to be. Then you realize that it is not their fault and things happen. They did not choose to become ill, but it has happened. Then you are filled with guilt because you feel such anger toward them. It becomes a vicious circle that plays out over and over again.

You are afraid of things yet to come.

Will you run out of money? Will you be able to keep this up? How are you going to lift him in and out of bed or the bathtub?

These are just some of the thoughts that you might have on a regular basis.

Yes, being a caregiver can be lonely and stressful, we know. Tens of millions share your experience. The sheer number of people aging in our society today tells us that the number of caregivers is only going to rise exponentially too.

And while the challenges of being a caregiver are immense, they can be met. Our goal is to give you the tools you need to do just that.

Think of reading this book like going to the gym. With exercise, weights don't get any lighter. But over time the weighty burden *feels* lighter as you get stronger.

Our goal is to help you get stronger as a caregiver. We want:

To encourage you

You have permission to feel the way you do when things look bleak. And, know that it will pass, and things will get better. You can do this. You will make it.

To let you know you are not alone

You are not alone. There are millions of people, just like you, living as caregivers right now. Others suffer in silence as you may do. Chances are you know several of them, but you just may not have had a chance to connect with any of them yet to share stories and help each other through.

To give you the strength to carry on when you feel like giving up

There will be days and nights that you will feel like giving up. It happens to all of us. It's normal. It may be small and seem insignificant at the time, but something will happen to cheer you up and pick you up. Celebrate and hold onto the small and simple victories and happy times to get you through the more challenging times.

To give you the practical tools you need to make it through each day the best you can

Each chapter of this book will end with Things to Do Now, practical steps to help you implement the principles discussed. Because we don't just want to inspire you. We want to inspire you to act in a way that will make a positive difference, for you and those you love and care for.

Here's what we'll cover in the following chapters:

- Why taking care of yourself first is paramount

- How to manage your guilt and anger

- How to think differently to act differently

- How to deal with small, daily changes

- How to deal with big, life-altering changes

- How to ask for help and be okay with it

- How to pursue your path to happiness

Being a caregiver is a journey. We're happy to walk that journey with you.

Chapter One

Put Your Mask on First

If we lose cabin pressure, oxygen masks will drop ... If you are traveling with someone who needs assistance, put your mask on first.

The implication of this warning given at the beginning of every airline flight is clear:

- To help others you care for, you have to take care for yourself first.

So too for caregivers:

- *You cannot take care of loved ones long-term, if you do not take care of yourself short-term.*

It is okay to take care of yourself, even if it is only for a few minutes each day. You have permission, and we encourage you to take care of yourself. Every month, every week, every day, carve out some time to renew and refresh. Whether it is making sure that you eat, or get some sleep, or just have a few minutes to sit down and enjoy some solitude, take care of yourself first. If you do not, you run the risk of wearing yourself out, becoming run-down, or becoming sick yourself, which will help no one in the end. Part of putting your mask on first is learning to ask for help too.

Some of the most challenging decisions a caregiver faces are (1) to accept the help that someone is offering or (2) to admit that you need it and to ask for help. The reasons can vary: You do not trust someone to do the job as well as you can; you feel guilty for "leaving" your loved one; or you feel like you are letting yourself down by admitting you need help.

Whatever the reason, we encourage you to figure out what will work for you to justify accepting help. That's part of putting your mask on first.

Superman and Wonder Woman are make-believe characters. We all wish and hope we could be them, but we aren't. Please realize that no one can be a full-time, family caregiver all by themselves. We all need help from time to time.

Let's look at this a couple of different ways:

1. Let's say before you became a caregiver, you worked for 40 years at a local grocery store. You worked your way up to management over the years. While you were there, you worked a minimum of 40 hours per week. Often you would put in 50 or 60 hours per week because you were either asked to, or the job just required it. At the end of each day though, when it finally ended, you were able to go home and spend time with your family. You went bowling every Wednesday night and had the opportunity to get a good night's sleep most nights. The bottom line is, you had time for you.

Now, however, you don't go to work outside the home every day, but you are on call 24 hours a day, seven days a week in the home. There is no store or office to go to during the day, and no separate home to go to at night or on the weekends. Your loved one lives with you, and you are the one who is there to help them if the need is there to do the following: get dressed, prepare breakfast, lunch, and dinner, feed them, get them to the doctor, help them bathe, or calm them down.

But there is no one there for you. And things can happen without a warning or notice. You could be sitting down to enjoy a well-deserved cup of tea while your loved one starts a nap, only to let the tea sit and get cold because your loved one was calling for help to get to the toilet. Sound familiar?

2. You are working full-time as the office manager of a small company. You work

on operation items, HR issues as they arise, customer service, and collections as needed. In essence you handle many different issues and work with many different people every day, and the pace is non-stop. You work 40 hours per week, and by the end of each day and each week, you are tired and look forward to going home. But the "going home" is now starting to get challenging as well. One year ago, you began to help your father a few nights per week as his dementia began to progress. This evolved into a daily visit to his house for a few hours before going home to yours.

As the dementia progressed even further, you and your partner decided to have your father come live with you. Your partner helps out as much as possible, but travels during the week, so for the most part you are on your own Monday through Friday.

As the weeks turn into months, you start to worry more and more about your father being home alone during the day. Little worries pop in your head: "Is he safe?" "What is he doing?" "Is he using the stove to heat up food?" "Will he remember to turn it off when he is done?" Your stress and worry are replacing your smiles and laughter, and you are noticing how you have less patience now, and you are becoming more easily frustrated at work.

The day's events are fast paced and never stop. It seems like you are trying to fit more and more into each day but somehow it is never enough. Something's going to give. Please make sure it is not you.

Perhaps you can start the process of taking care of you by committing, for their benefit and yours, to putting your mask on first. If not, and you get sick, you will not be able to care for you or your loved one either.

We know this is easier said than done.
It's tough when you have to:

- Be a doctor, nurse, cheerleader, parent, defender, cook, maid, butler, and superhero all wrapped into one.

- Live on coffee and junk food and struggle to stay awake because you had three nights of little sleep, because your loved one was hallucinating or having bad dreams throughout the previous nights.

- Drive to doctor appointments, drugstores, and grocery stores.

- Try to keep the house and your clothes clean, and take care of all the other little daily chores that can stack up.

Still, it's important to find a way to take care of you first. It's like the story author Stephen Covey used to tell:

A man speeding down the highway was running very low on gas. "Shouldn't you pull over and fill up your tank?" his companion asked. "I don't have time to pull over and fill up," the man responded. "I have to get to where I'm going!"

We can all smile at the obvious end result of such thinking. Yet when it comes to our own reality, it's easy to think and act like that man from time to time:

- We drive so hard to get someplace, that we lose sight of the fact we are about to run out of gas.

Yet that's exactly what may happen if you don't take the time to fill up your tank. So we encourage you to commit to putting your mask on first.

- Remember: In order to take care of them, you have to take care of you!

Let's look at another example of real consequences that can happen if you do not take care of you.

8

Let's say you have been a full-time caregiver for your wife, Susan, for the past three years. She has dementia, and things have really progressed the past 12 months. She does not recognize you all the time. You are diabetic and have high blood pressure too.

A neighbor, whom you have known for years, knows the situation you are in. She has offered to come over on Thursdays to sit with Susan, so you can make a weekly trip to the grocery store when they offer a 5% discount for senior citizens. You accept the offer because Susan has always been comfortable with your neighbor. They used to go for coffee regularly, and your wife always enjoyed her company.

Besides, other than the neighbor, you realize that there is no other immediate help for you. Your kids all live out of state and have their own families. You do not want to burden them with your troubles.

The past few months you have really appreciated your neighbor's help, since taking your wife out has become more and more challenging for you.

One Thursday morning, you are anxious for your neighbor to come over as you are out of milk and several food staples. The week before you had to rush through the grocery store because your neighbor was sick, and you had your wife with you, and she was having a bad day. You rushed through the store then and were not able to get the normal food stocks because you just wanted to get Susan home.

This particular day, you keep glancing at the clock waiting for 10:00 a.m. to roll around, and at 9:59, your phone rings, and not your doorbell. It is your neighbor. She is still sick and will not be able to come over. Your heart drops as you were looking forward to a little alone time and to replenishing the pantry. You have not eaten well yourself the past few days and are beginning to "feel" it.

So you decide to go to the store, thinking you will just zip in and out as quickly as you can. You get Susan dressed and ready to go with you because leaving her at home alone is not feasible.

You get to the store and face a decision so many caregivers have: "Do I leave my adult loved one with dementia in the car so I can just run in and out, or do I take the extra time and potential headaches of getting her in and out of the car to go in with me?"

On sunny comfortable days, you usually take her in. On cold and/or rainy days, you usually let her stay in the car. Some days it is an easy decision, and other days it fills you with anguish trying to decide what is best.

It is stunning that just a few years ago you would have never given a trip to the grocery store a second thought, but today it has become a source of angst and difficult emotions and decisions.

Being a caregiver is like riding a daily roller coaster. You have to be physically and mentally fit to continue to care for the one you love. You will likely experience emotions ranging from joy to grief, from worry to relief. There will be small, simple victories to relish and small daily challenges to overcome.

The rest of this book is dedicated to helping you meet those challenges.

Five Things to Do Now to Help Put Your Mask on First:

1. **Small daily doses:** Take daily mini-vacations. A mini-vacation may mean reading your favorite magazine while your loved one naps. It may mean taking in some fresh air when you go out to get the mail. It may mean taking time to pray or meditate before you get up. Perhaps it means closing your eyes and taking some deep, soothing breaths in the physician's waiting room. Maybe it's listening to your favorite music as you drive to the store. The day is filled with opportunities for small moments of relaxation. Look for them and take advantage.

Top 10 "Daily Mini-Vacations" I will take:

_____

_____

_____

_____

_____

_____

_____

_____

_____

_____

_____

_____

_____

_____

_____

_____

_____

2. **Ask for, and accept, help:** If you feel like you are having trouble getting everything done, that's because it's hard to get it all done. It's not because something is wrong with you or you're not doing it right. Being a caregiver is hard. Most caregivers feel unprepared and overwhelmed, especially at first. That's normal.

Don't be shy asking for help. Many family members, friends, and neighbors want to help. Let them, and try to arrange back-up help in case they cannot make it on a particular day. Ask your doctor about support groups. Call your local senior center for information and referral sources for help. Try out different groups, services, and agencies before things reach a crisis point. It's not a sign of weakness to ask for help. It is a sign of wisdom and strength. You would want to be there for others who might need your help. Let them be there for you now. (More on this in Chapter Six.)

Who will I look to for help?

_____

_____

_____

_____

_____

_____

_____

_____

_____

_____

_____

_____

_____

_____

_____

_____

_____

3. **Stay in the moment:** The easiest way to stress out is to be doing one thing while you are worrying about six other things you need to do too. Train yourself to stay in the moment and focus on doing one thing at a time. Multi-tasking is not the way to go. You can do 10 things in an hour, but not 10 things at once. Break chores down into doable chunks, and do them one at a time.

Ways I will stay in the moment and focus:

_____

_____

_____

_____

_____

_____

_____

_____

4. **The basics of eating and sleeping:**
   This one is so basic it almost seems silly
   to mention. But often it is the easiest
   and simplest things we tend to neglect.
   So, make sure to eat to maintain your
   energy. This may mean 4-5 smaller
   meals over the course of the day with
   a focus on protein, versus 1-2 larger
   meals heavy on carbohydrates.
   Educate yourself on nutrition. There
   are multiple resources to choose from
   such as books, videos, your local
   senior center, or a food bank. Your
   doctor's office might also have
   information on healthy eating which
   they can provide you.

   Also, studies repeatedly show the
   importance of sleep for good mental
   and physical health. Most people need
   6-8 hours a night. Figure out how much
   sleep you need, and stick to it as best as
   possible. We know this can be a
   challenge if your loved one is having a
   bad night or if they sleep during the day
   and are up at night. You have to figure

out a schedule that works for you, and be able to accept assistance when it is offered so you can sleep.

Steps to remind myself to eat and sleep:

_____

_____

_____

_____

_____

_____

_____

_____

_____

_____

_____

_____

5. **Adopt an "all or something" mentality.** Maybe you can't do all of the things we suggest here. But you can do some of them. Start small. Pick one thing—reading a book, stepping out for a breath of fresh air and listening to the birds, and build from there. All those little "somethings" add up.

My "All or Something" Top Five:

_____

_____

_____

_____

_____

_____

_____

_____

_____

_____

Chapter Two

Dealing with Guilt and Anger

Eventually, most caregivers ask similar questions:

- Why did this happen to the one I love?
- Why did this happen to me?
- Why did this happen to *us*?

These thoughts are normal. They are expected. They happen to almost everyone at some point. You can never predict the exact situation that will trigger them, but next, let's look at some common scenarios.

Scenario 1: You as Your Spouse's Caregiver.

You did not plan on becoming a caregiver. Your plan was to retire and enjoy the Golden Years with your loved one—travel, spend time with the kids and grandkids, sleep in, and go out with friends.

You were going to do whatever you wanted to do because you could.

The only problem is no one told the Golden Years that was the plan. Your loved one was not supposed to be sick. You were not supposed to be a caregiver. Sometimes it feels like the term Golden Years is just an ongoing joke. We each see the punch line at different times, and we each feel like we are the only ones who see it.

Scenario 2: You as The Sandwich Generation Caregiver

You are not alone in this double caregiving effort. At the time of this book's printing:

- Just over 1 of every 8 Americans aged 40 to 60 is both raising a child and caring for a parent.

- Between 7 to 10 million adults are caring for their aging parents from long distance.

Chances are very good that many of these Sandwich Generation caregivers are also working a full-time job as well.

You are "sandwiched" between your parent, your kids, and possibly your career. This can be coupled with role reversal in both directions as well: You were once taken care of by your parents, but you are now tasked with taking care of them.

Your parents are either on their own and need assistance with things like household chores, repairs, and maybe some assistance with paperwork; or they live with you as a result of an illness. You are somewhere in the middle of that, trying to find balance.

Often there is a financial burden too—trying to assist parents with their income or money management, while trying to assist children paying off their student loans and starting their lives—it can all be overwhelming.

It can also lead to common questions you may have asked yourself: "Will this ever end? And, what about me and my dreams? Are they gone forever?"

All of this can trigger common but often uncomfortable emotions: primarily guilt and anger. The fact is, we all experience anger and guilt at times. It's called being human. And many caregivers also know the feeling of complete isolation and offering up the prayer of, "Lord, if you are really up there, please help me get through this day."

We want you to know, it is okay to feel all that. In fact, it's more than okay. It's normal to react emotionally to the situations you find yourself in.

Consider the following, and see if it resonates with you somehow: One night, your loved one is having a bad night and tries to get up and move around the house because of a bad dream. After you finally get them calmed down and back to sleep, you are wide awake. Your adrenaline is flowing, and you only had what amounted to a 60-minute power nap before the episode with your loved one started.

You cannot get back to sleep, so you turn on the TV and start flipping channels. You find a movie that you love but have not seen in years. As you are watching, you realize that the first time you saw this movie was on your first date with your loved one, when the world and your lives were ahead of you. You start thinking about all of the things you did back then and the plans you had to make a life together; to have a family, and then travel the world and enjoy retirement.

Unfortunately, your personal movie and dreams got cut short because of an unanticipated illness. And then, those "Why did this have to happen?" questions started.

Often, those questions can stir up anger as well. That too is normal and to be expected.

Does your thinking about your loved one ever sometimes go like this?

- Why are you so demanding?

- Can't you see I'm trying to help?

- Why can't you show more appreciation?

- Can't you see that I have sacrificed everything for you?

Those thoughts can trigger anger. And then, on top of it all, anger can often quite quickly be followed by guilt.

The guilt may come from thoughts like these:

- Who am I to question God/fate?

- My loved one did not ask for this. Why am I mad at them?

- Life happens. Why can't I just accept that this is what's happened?

Finally, the guilt and anger may culminate in this:

- *I shouldn't feel this way!*

Here's what we hope you will come
to realize:

- There is no one way everyone
  should feel.
- No two people feel exactly the
  same way when faced with
  similar situations.
- Everyone feels what they feel,
  and that's okay.
- It's what *you do* in response to
  your thoughts and feelings that
  matters most.

For example:

- Talking out your thoughts and feelings
  with a trusted advisor or friend?
  That's good.
- Holding feelings in, blaming yourself
  and/or others, or exploding in angry
  outbursts? Not so good.

It is also important to note in that latter
example, that even when an angry outburst

does not involve yelling or raising your voice, it may be an issue if your loved one sees or senses it.

78% of our communication is nonverbal. What does that mean to you? It means that your loved one can probably read you like a book.

If you are angry and your body language shows it, it still can be very bad for both of you. Your loved one may mirror your mood, which can lead to a very stressful and angry day for you both.

Having feelings isn't a problem. It's how you choose to act on them that counts the most.

And finally, it's probably important to feel *something.* Because to feel, is to be human.

If you feel nothing on the outside, it's possible you are holding something in on the inside, and that's not usually a good thing.

Holding strong feelings in can sometimes be associated with things like:

- Depression
- Anxiety
- Headaches
- Other emotional or physical problems

You may want to think about it like this: Do you remember the last day that you were not feeling well or had a splitting headache? Did that make it easier or harder to accomplish the daily caregiving tasks such as cooking, bathing, or getting to the doctor's office? So, if you can find a way to let go of the feelings of anger or guilt to minimize any negative consequence, please do it.

You can think of guilt and anger as two sides of the same coin: Each emotion may trigger the other.

While guilt and anger often go together, it does not mean they have to *go on* indefinitely. They will pass, if you let them.

Below are five tips on how to manage the emotions that often go along with being a caregiver.

Five Ways to Manage Guilt and Anger

1. **Reframe guilt and anger as normal.** To be human is to feel. And to be a caregiver is to feel guilt and anger at some point. When you feel these things, remind yourself that this is normal. But that does not mean you have to be a slave to your feelings. Sometimes changing our thinking can change how we feel. When you find yourself in a negative pattern of self-talk, see if you can counter that with a more positive thought.

   Top five ways to change my thinking to change feelings:

   _____

   _____

   _____

   _____

_____

_____

_____

_____

_____

_____

_____

_____

_____

_____

_____

_____

_____

_____

_____

_____

_____

2. **Find someone to talk it out.** Talking about feelings often helps to relieve them. Find someone you can trust, and bounce your thoughts and feelings off them. Your confidant can be a close friend, family member, or sometimes a person removed from your situation who may have a clearer perspective. This may be a clergy member or a professional counselor. Ask your health care professional if there are support groups for folks going though similar experiences.

Who I can talk to about my problems?

_____

_____

_____

_____

_____

_____

_____

3. **Journaling.** Sometimes writing down your thoughts and feelings can be an effective way of coping with them. This may be especially true if you are a more private person, or feel too uncomfortable talking with others about your innermost thoughts and feelings. Keep a journal and write in it every day. Write down what happened that day and how you thought and felt about it. Share your hopes and dreams and fears. Getting negative feelings out in this manner may rob them of their power. And writing down positive feelings can bring them to life. This is for your eyes only so write whatever you wish. No need to hold back.

When, where, and how
I will journal—(pen and paper,
blog, etc.):

_____

_____

_____

_____

_____

_____

_____

_____

_____

_____

_____

_____

_____

_____

_____

_____

_____

_____

_____

_____

_____

_____

4. **Listen to music.** Listening to music is a great way to release feelings and emotion. Play your favorite artist, and listen to your favorite pieces. Whether you relate to the words, or the melody, or both, let the music wash over you while it washes the emotions out. Music can be the emotional equivalent of taking a shower. You will feel clean and refreshed afterward.

My favorite songs:

_____

_____

_____

_____

_____

My favorite singers:

_____

_____

_____

_____

5. **Pray and/or learn to meditate.**
If you are a religious person, lean on your faith for support. Pray and read scripture. Learning to meditate may help too, whether you are particularly religious or not. Meditation is nothing more than a way to quiet your mind and body. It's an excellent way to manage stress.

My favorite prayers:

_____

_____

_____

_____

Places I can quietly meditate:

_____

_____

_____

_____

_____

_____

_____

_____

_____

_____

_____

_____

_____

_____

_____

_____

_____

_____

_____

_____

_____

_____

Chapter Three

A Simple Model
for Dealing with Change

To deal with change, it helps to understand why we do what we do.

Human behavior often follows this simple pattern:

Think—Feel—Do—Get

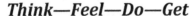

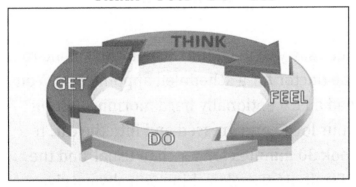

- What you think, triggers what you feel

- What you feel, triggers what you do

- What you do, triggers what you get, both in terms of what you get to accomplish on the outside, and what you get to experience on the inside

For example, let's say you go to a doctor you do not particularly like. You had a bad experience before and now you think like this:

"I don't like this doctor or his staff. He never listens to me about what's wrong, and they all seem hurried and harried all the time."

Now that you have a dislike of that doctor and his staff, let's add another layer and look at it from a slightly different angle.

Let's say you need to take your loved one to the doctor for a scheduled appointment. You had an exceptionally hard morning getting your loved one dressed and into the car. It took 30 minutes longer than usual, and the 45-minute travel cushion you always give yourself is almost gone. You finally get to the doctor's office and your loved one does not want to get out of the car. They do not recognize the building, and they think you are lying to them about where they are and about what is going to happen next. It takes another 20 minutes to get them into the doctor's office, and now you are officially late. The receptionist takes your name and points out the obvious in a snotty tone— you are late.

You think to yourself, "I know we are late. Who are you to talk to me that way? Do you have any idea what it is like being a caregiver? Do you know what I go through every day?"

These thoughts trigger your anxiety and anger. Your anxiety and anger, like pouring gas on a fire, fuel your impatience. Perhaps you don't smile and are more abrupt than usual. Maybe you make a snide comment to yourself under your breath. The staff picks up on that and things go downhill from there. A bad experience is made worse.

Here's the deal:

If you want things to change, you have to change. And when *you* change, you have a chance to influence those around you to change too.

For example, what if you tried changing the pattern by thinking like this?

"Being late is not the end of the world. I did the best I could, so I'll cut myself some slack. Guess these folks have a tough job too. Glad I don't have to do what they do all day. Think I'll kill 'em with kindness this time around."

Remember, you get more with an ounce of sugar than you do a pound of vinegar. These thoughts calm you down. Your tone and body language are more pleasant when you arrive at the office. Maybe the staff picks up on this and responds in kind.

And maybe not.

You can't *control* anyone else's behavior. But everything you do can *influence* someone else's behavior.

Don't you have a better chance of influencing better behavior in them, through better behavior yourself?

Even if they don't respond as you might wish, *you* still get to experience being calm and in control.

Isn't that better than letting someone else dictate how you will feel throughout your day?

Another principle is at play here: *You always get what you give.*

For example, if you give someone a hard time, you get to experience a hard time. Or, if you give someone love, you get to experience love.

You always experience what you give to others, *regardless of what they give back to you.*

Why not always give what you want to experience?

Would it help if we said it this way?

Treat others as you want them to treat you.

Finally, there are two kinds of change:

1. Change you can see coming from a distance, like a far-off train. For example, we can predict some of the changes that come with age: decreased muscle tone or perhaps a slight loss in hearing, and "Where did I put my glasses!"

2. The sudden change that seems to come out of nowhere and may run you over: the out-of-nowhere stuff that includes things like accidents, heart attacks, sudden illnesses, etc.

Both types of change are stressful. In the next few chapters we will explore how to deal with that stress to get the outcomes that you want.

Five Things to Do Now to Make Simple Changes for Lasting Impact

1. **Inner Voice:** Pay attention to that little voice in the back of your head. We all have that voice. Like a color

commentator calling a sporting event, it's always there in the background, commenting on the action going on. The voice is so common and continuous we may not even notice it's there, but it always is. If that voice is adding joy to your world, great. If it is adding stress, change what it says.

Thoughts I will use to counteract the little voice when it turns negative:

_____

_____

_____

_____

_____

_____

_____

_____

_____

_____

2. **Watch Your Triggers:** It's important to
   pay attention to that voice because
   often it is the first thought that triggers
   the think—feel—do—get cycle. For
   example, let's say you wake up and
   notice it's raining. The voice says, "Ugh,
   what an ugly day. This weather is
   horrible." Well, you've just set yourself
   up for a horrible day. The negative
   voice triggers negative feelings and
   you're off to the negative races.

*Past examples of negative
first thoughts that I can change into
positive ones in the future:*

_____

_____

_____

_____

_____

_____

_____

_____

_____

_____

_____

_____

_____

_____

_____

_____

_____

_____

_____

_____

_____

_____

_____

_____

_____

3. **Stop Your Negativity**: When you catch your voice setting you up for negative consequences, change it. After all, it's your voice! So, for example, if you wake up and notice it's raining, why not say to yourself, "What a beautiful rain. We certainly need it. Thank God for the rain."

Steps I will take to change a negative thought to a positive. I am the only one who can do it!

_____

_____

_____

_____

_____

_____

_____

_____

_____

4. What Part of You Will You Listen to?

It is true that both voices are made up. That is, they are *add-ons* to the fact that it is raining. But which voice is likely to trigger more upbeat emotions and behavior and outcomes?

Which voice will I listen to?
I am the only one who knows!

_____

_____

_____

_____

_____

_____

_____

_____

_____

_____

_____

_____

5. **Create Uplifting Messages:**
Remember, that voice is yours. Becoming aware of what you tell yourself is step one. Telling yourself uplifting messages is step two. Then repeat. Often.

Messages I can give myself early and often to stay positive.
I am the only one who knows!

_____

_____

_____

_____

_____

_____

_____

_____

_____

_____

_____

Chapter Four

Dealing with
Small Daily Changes

Being a caregiver is hard because, well, it's hard. It's not hard because you aren't doing it right. There are no magic formulas or silver bullets to make everything go smoothly all the time.

As your loved one's medical issues progress, your loved one will likely continue to change behaviorally too. Physical and cognitive abilities may diminish. Their ability to have a conversation, or bathe, or feed themselves may disappear.

For an adult child, it can be challenging emotionally the first time you bathe your parent. You can and should read about it, prepare for it, and plan it, but there is still an emotional shock getting used to bathing the person that raised and bathed you.

To help you better deal with these small daily changes, it can be helpful to distinguish between problems and dilemmas. This helpful concept was developed by a leadership consultant named Jonno Hanafin[1].

According to Hanafin:

Problems have solutions.

- For example, if the lightbulb is out, change it.
- If the car breaks down, repair it.
- If you are out of toilet paper, buy some more.

Dilemmas are situations with conflicting forces that by definition *have no solution.*

- For example, you need time for yourself, but your loved one needs care 24/7.
- Treatment for one medical condition makes another condition worse.

- Your doctors and pharmacists are not always on the same page. They give you important, but contradictory advice.

Unlike problems, there are no solutions for dilemmas. All you can do is manage them, and balance the conflicting forces the best you can.

The distinction between problems and dilemmas is important. Here's why:

- If you try to solve a dilemma, you will drive yourself crazy because there is no solution.
- If you try to manage a problem—say trying to tell all the doctors and pharmacists what to do—you will drive everybody else crazy. They are not likely to listen anyway.

A caregiver's day is filled with both problems and dilemmas. Identifying which is which and then acting accordingly can help lower your stress and increase your effectiveness on a day-to-day basis. Solving the problems and managing the dilemmas is the best way to go.

Another thing to try and avoid, if you can, is turning smaller problems into bigger ones. A phrase that may be helpful here is, "What is, is."

For instance, let's say your hot water heater goes, and there is no hot water in the house. That's the reality. That's what is. You can fuss and fume and lay the blame, or you can pick up the phone and call a plumber. Which of these responses is likely to solve the problem best?

Yes, it may feel good occasionally to kick and scream if you will, to get something off your chest. But if you find yourself constantly holding on to ways of thinking and feeling that only end up holding you down or holding you back, you may want to reconsider your approach.

In sum, managing the small daily challenges really comes down to managing yourself to get the results that you want. Following are some tips to help you do just that.

Five Things to Try Now to Manage Small Daily Changes

1. **List all of your daily activities.** Start below or get a separate piece of paper and divide it into two columns. If it is a problem with a clear solution (even if you are not sure what the solution is yet), place it in the left-hand column or below.

Challenging Daily Activities— Problems:

_____

_____

_____

_____

_____

_____

_____

_____

_____

_____

_____

_____

_____

_____

_____

_____

_____

If you think the change is a dilemma that has many possible ways to approach it, place it in the right-hand column on your separate piece of paper or below.

Challenging Daily Activities— Dilemmas:

_____

_____

_____

_____

2. **Next, map out how you will solve that day's problems.** For example, if you are out of supplies, plan when you will go to the store. Or ask a friend to run an errand. If you need to change an appointment, make the call and pick a new date and time.

Solutions to Your Problems:

_____

_____

_____

_____

_____

_____

_____

_____

_____

_____

_____

_____

3. **Strategize how to manage the dilemmas.** This might involve conversations with others and making difficult trade-offs and decisions. For example, treating one condition may create less than desirable side effects. You and your loved one will have to choose whether the treatment is worth the risk. Managing dilemmas is about choosing the lesser of two evils sometimes.

Best Ways to Manage My Dilemmas:

_____

_____

_____

_____

_____

_____

_____

_____

_____

_____

_____

_____

_____

_____

_____

_____

_____

_____

_____

_____

_____

_____

_____

_____

_____

_____

4. **Don't be afraid to ask for help in either solving problems or managing dilemmas.** Let those who want to help, help.

Who will you ask for help—For Tasks?

_____

_____

_____

_____

_____

_____

_____

_____

_____

_____

_____

_____

_____

Who would you feel comfortable talking to about your dilemmas?

_____

_____

_____

_____

_____

_____

_____

_____

_____

_____

_____

_____

_____

_____

5. **And don't forget to Put Your Mask on First!**

   Small things I will do today to take care of me:

   _____

   _____

   _____

   _____

   _____

   _____

   _____

   _____

   _____

   _____

   _____

   _____

   _____

Chapter Five

Dealing with Big, Life-Altering Change

Rarely do we enter relationships knowing that being a caregiver will become a focal point of the relationship.

But sometimes it happens:

- A child is born deathly ill

- A family member comes down with a chronic disease

- An accident turns your world (and theirs) upside down

With such change comes sudden loss:

- Loss of the life we had in the present

- Loss of the life we envisioned

- Loss of the life we once knew

We don't ask for changes like these.

Yet they may happen. The stress and strain can go far beyond the disruption of daily routines.

Life-altering change can disrupt your sense of self. It can cause you to question all that you know: about you, others, God, and life in general. It may challenge your faith. Stress may disrupt relationships to the breaking point at times.

If any of this describes you or sounds familiar, *please know you are not alone.*

Others have learned how to adapt and cope. You can too.

It's true that there are no magic bullets to make all this go away. And you can't go backward in time. But you can go forward.

It's how you choose to go forward that can make all the difference.

Here are some tips to help get you moving in the right direction.

First, give yourself time. Change may come suddenly, but adapting to it takes time.

You may well experience some or all of the five stages of grief:

1. Denial. The first stage may involve disbelief. Sometimes the mind reacts to overwhelming change by denying the change has happened.

2. Anger. Once the denial wears off, anger often kicks in. That's where the questions we covered in Chapter Two may occur: "Why me? Why us? Why did this have to happen? It's not fair!"

3. Bargaining. In this stage, people often bargain with a higher power to change the outcome: "If you just let them be healed or make things go differently, I promise to ..."

4. Depression. A sense of loss and hopelessness may kick in when you sense that bargaining has not worked to change the situation.

5. Acceptance. At this stage you are ready to let go of what was, so you can latch on to what is.

Know that these stages are normal for many people experiencing loss. Not everyone goes through every stage or in the same order, but most go through something that resembles these stages.

Second, to deal with loss, it can help to learn to let go.

Let us explain. It is hard to begin a new life by holding on to your old life. If you continue to think about and focus your energies on what was, you will have less energy and attention for the realities of now. Learning to let go of the past by changing your thoughts and feelings can be helpful. At the end of this chapter, we will offer some tips on how to do so.

Third, it can be easier to let go if you learn how to latch on too. Specifically, we encourage you to mentally latch on to what has *not* changed: *primarily your love and devotion to your loved one.*

Other things that change cannot affect:

- Other's love for you

- Your fundamental values and beliefs

- Your love for others

In summary, often you cannot control change in your life. But you can always choose your response. Latching on to what has not changed, can help you cope with what has.

Five Things to Try Now for Dealing with Big, Life-Altering Change:

1. **Make a list of all the things in your life that have not changed.** These may include your values, love, and whatever matters most in the deepest recesses of your heart.

What has not changed in my life?

_____

_____

_____

_____

_____

_____

_____

_____

_____

_____

_____

_____

_____

_____

_____

_____

_____

_____

_____

_____

_____

_____

_____

2. **Journal about the things that have changed, and write down your feelings about them.**

Will you commit to journaling about the things that have changed in your life?

I, _____,
commit myself to writing about the things that have changed in my life since I became a caregiver and how they make me feel.

_____   _____

Signature   Date

3. **Routines.** As quickly as possible, establish a new routine. This will become your new normal.

What are the items in my routine that can be changed immediately?

_____

_____

_____

_____

_____

_____

_____

_____

_____

_____

_____

_____

_____

4. **Re-read Chapter One** about putting your mask on first. It's time to maintain your stamina and well-being as best you can.

5. **Goals.** Establishing new goals and putting yourself on a path to achieving them is a good way to let go of the past to embrace the future.

   What are my new goals?

   _____

   _____

   _____

   _____

   _____

   _____

   _____

   _____

   _____

How will I achieve my goals?

_____

_____

_____

_____

_____

_____

_____

_____

_____

_____

_____

_____

_____

_____

_____

_____

Chapter Six

How to Ask for Help

Asking for help can be hard. Heck, many men don't even want to ask for directions, much less ask for help in being a caregiver! Of course, the same can be true for women too.

Sometimes asking for help makes us feel weak. It might make us feel we aren't as strong as we should be, or we somehow just aren't doing it right.

Let us make this as clear as we can:

There is no right way to be a caregiver!

But there is *your way* to be a caregiver, and that's what we hope you are discovering as you are reading this book. Hopefully you are discovering what works for you and your loved one. Please do not doubt yourself. Recognize that you are now *the* expert in caregiving for your loved one.

Freeing Yourself of *Have To's,* *Should's,* and *Ought's*

If we're not careful, life can become full of *Have To's, Should's,* and *Ought's.* That little voice we discussed earlier can tell us that no matter what we are doing at any particular moment, we *should* be doing this, we *ought* to be doing that. Or, I *have to* do this and that, etc.

And, when it comes to asking for help, that little voice might say something like this: "I *shouldn't* have to ask for help. I *ought* to be able to do this on my own. I *have to* figure this out on my own."

And the items on the little voice's list can add up. The list of *Should's* and *Ought's* might contain many major items or many little items that build up on a mental checklist. The list can become overwhelming because you think you *have to, should,* and *ought* to do those things right away.

And when you don't, the little voice may double down and say even louder: "YOU *SHOULD* BE ABLE TO DO ALL THIS! YOU *HAVE TO!*"

The everyday *Have To's* could be as simple as:

- I *have to* wash the floor.

- I *have to* clean that spot on the carpet.

- I *have to* get to the grocery store to get more laundry detergent to wash the sheets because we are *almost* out of detergent.

Maybe you were not able to get to these *Have To's* right away because the caregiver you scheduled to come in did not make it, or you were so exhausted when they came that you needed to take a nap.

The practical *Should's* could be things like:

- I *should* caulk the windows to help reduce the gas and electric bills.

- I *should* get the leaves off of the ground so they don't blow into the house when I let the dogs in and out.

- I *should* get to the store to buy a new filter for the air conditioner because it is time to change it.

These are on your to do list. The moment you think about doing them, your loved one is having a bad day, and you cannot get anything else done but attend to your loved one.

The *Ought's* could be things like:

- I *ought* to paint the shed in the backyard because it is chipping.

- I *ought* to rearrange the linen closet to make it easier to get the sheets and towels in and out.

- I *ought* to paint the hallway walls because he keeps banging his walker into the walls and leaving marks.

Maybe these are things that you had never done in your life because your loved one always did them. You know you can do it, in fact, you want to. But as the list of things you *ought* to do keeps growing, so do the personal needs of your loved one. You spend more time with them and have no free time for the *Ought's*.

Filling your mind with *Have To's*, *Should's*, and *Ought's* will only add to your stress. Being a caregiver is stressful enough without piling on other issues for you to worry about.

A colleague of ours once suggested, don't *should* all over yourself! Instead of thinking, "I *should* do this," or "I *ought* to do that," or "I *have to* do this," think, "What do I *want* to do right now?"

True, maybe what you want to do right now is sit down and read the paper, but it's time to feed your loved one, or to get them dressed, or any other myriad duties one is called to do as a caregiver.

But at least you can think of it as, "Yes, I'd like to read the paper right now, but I also want to take care of my loved one, so I'll do that now. I'll get back to my paper as soon as I can."

Remember, how we think triggers what we feel. If your thoughts are about what you *have to* do, or *ought* to do, or *should* do are triggering more stress than anything else, then perhaps it is time to change those thoughts.

Let's use our previous example of, "I *have to* get to the store to buy detergent because we are almost out," and try looking at it this way:

First you are *almost* out, which means you probably have enough for a load or two of laundry. Second, you have been shopping at the same store for years, and you take pride in the fact that you can get a week's worth of groceries picked out and paid for in 20 minutes. Those two things combined give you the opportunity to take advantage of your friend's offer to help. You can have them come over while your loved one is down for a nap. You can run to the store and be back in time to share a cup of coffee with your friend while your loved one is still napping.

And, you might want to add:

"And, I want to take care of myself and put my mask on first. I've been going at it hard now for eight days straight. I have had offers of help. Maybe I am going to accept those offers and schedule a day and time for my neighbor to come over, so I can take a walk, or take a nap, or grab a sandwich at the diner down the street, because a sandwich always seems to taste better when I don't *have to* make it myself."

Another thought that can stop us from asking for help or from accepting help that is offered is this: "I don't want to be a bother to anyone."

This is a *BIGGIE*. Many of us don't want to feel like we are burdening others, whether they are friends, family, acquaintances from our place of worship, or from some other social connection in the community.

Here's the thing: If people offer to help, that means they want to. You aren't burdening them. You are doing what they want. You are helping them feel like they are making a difference because, well, they are.

We encourage you to assume that if someone offers to help, they mean it. So let them!

So:

- If the men from the synagogue want to organize a yard cleanup day for you— let them!

- If your neighbors want to provide some meals—let them!

- If someone from work wants to help with the driving—let them!

Have you ever thought about the fact that by letting others help you, that you are in fact helping them? That you are allowing them to make a contribution and feel like they are making a difference? Do you really want to rob others of this chance to feel good about themselves? We didn't think so.

Perhaps you have caught the mantra of this chapter:

If someone wants to help—let them!

This is a two-step acceptance strategy.

Step 1: Accept the help.

Remember if the roles were reversed, you would want to help your friends and family, so let them help you in your time of need.

Step 2: Get specific on the help right away.

If someone offers to go to the store and pick something up for you, get them the list immediately.

If someone offers to sit with your loved one for a couple of hours to give you a break, accept and schedule a day and time immediately. Schedule it whether you think you need it not. Why? Because life happens. You know as well as anyone that things can change at the drop of a hat, but life goes on.

Does this sound familiar? A neighbor offers to sit with your loved one so you can run errands anytime you need it. You thank them, and tell them you will take them up on their offer. A few days later, you call because you are having a tough time and need a break. Unfortunately, the neighbor is sick and cannot come over, or they took an unexpected trip out of town, or their air conditioner broke and they are waiting on the repairman.

Has this happened so many times that you have just stopped taking people up on their offers for help because you "know" they will not follow through, and they just do not mean it? Could this be one of the things that is causing you to feel so alone?

See if _Step 2_ of accepting someone's offer for help can change your life and theirs. Accept the offer and schedule times and days immediately. Be specific. Watch and see how you feel when you create a one-time scheduled visit and the neighbor shows up. Will you still feel so all alone? Will you begin to believe that others will help because they want to?

Remember, if the roles were reversed, you would offer to help your neighbor and have done it in years past. You meant it when you offered help then, didn't you?

When Your Loved One Wants to Help

As much as possible, for as long as possible, it's a good idea to let the loved one you care for help themselves as much as possible too. They don't want to be a burden either, and a sense of independence is important for us all.

For example, I remember a time when I was selling shoes in a mall shoe store. A family

came in—Mom, Dad, and two small kids.
Dad was in a wheelchair. He hung his head.
Mom did all the talking.

When I asked how I could help them, Mom
replied, "He would like some cowboy boots,"
nodding her head toward her husband.

I looked at him. "What kind of boots are you
interested in, sir?" His head still hung, and
he did not answer. "He wants such and such
kind of boots," Mom said.

Meanwhile the kids were running around
the store acting up. Mom and Dad were
ignoring them. I continued to look at
the dad.

"Are those the kind of boots you are
interested in, sir?" I said, pointing at
a display.

Finally, the dad perked up and began to
engage with me. We looked at a variety of
boots, and he finally decided on a pair he
was interested in.

"One problem," he said. "My legs are mostly paralyzed. I don't see how we can try them on."

"Well, I bet we can make that work," I said. "Let me help."

And he did let me help.

Together, we pulled and pushed and shoved until we got the boots on. They looked great.

Then, I noticed something really cool: Dad was no longer hanging his head. His wife was no longer speaking for him. He was looking me in the eye and speaking for himself.

He began to corral his kids and to tell them to knock it off and get in line, and they listened!

I'm not sure who felt better as they left the store: me for having had a chance to help and make a difference, or the smiling dad holding his head high as he rolled out the store with his family and his new boots!

Remember: If you let people help, you are offering them a gift—the gift of being of service to others.

True, not everyone has that gift or wants to be of service, but there are likely many more than you might believe. Let them be of service to you. You, they, and your loved one will be better for it.

Five Things to Try Now
to Let go of Your *Should's* and *Ought's*
and to Ask for Help:

1. **Make a list of all the people who have offered to help.** Think about what they might do to help you with logistics and help them feel better. Then reach out and accept their offer.

Who has offered to help?
Who are the "go to" people
you will accept help from?

_____

_____

_____

_____

_____

_____

_____

_____

_____

_____

_____

_____

_____

_____

2. **Spread the love around. Rather than being afraid to ask for help, ask *more* people for help.** That way, if you truly are concerned about being a burden, you can rest assured you won't be because no one person is responsible for doing too much.

Who else can help and what are the specific little items that each can help with?

_____

_____

_____

_____

_____

_____

_____

_____

_____

3. **Don't be afraid to ask family for help either, especially kids.** You need the help, and they need to learn the value of sacrifice for others, especially the younger ones. Help them learn that lesson.

What family members can get involved?

_____

_____

_____

_____

_____

_____

_____

_____

_____

_____

4. **Pay attention to that little voice in the back of your head we talked about in Chapter Three.** When it tells you, "Don't be a burden," try answering with, "I'm not. By the way, shut up! I'm letting others experience the gift of giving."

5. **Asking for help can make some of us feel uncomfortable, and that's okay.** Going to the gym makes us uncomfortable too, but that's why we go! Otherwise we accomplish nothing. Experiment allowing yourself to feel uncomfortable when asking for or accepting help. Rest assured it will get easier over time.

Chapter Seven

Pursuing Your
Path to Happiness

Throughout this book we have discussed some of the burdens being a caregiver can create and shared some ideas on how best to handle those burdens. We hope you have discovered that you are not alone in the burdens you face, and that you don't have to face them alone either.

We have encouraged you to recognize that being a caregiver is hard because it is hard. We have encouraged you to listen to that little voice in the back of your head, and tell it to "Shut up!" when it is only adding to your stress, not helping to reduce it.

We have encouraged you to replace negative thoughts with more positive ones whenever you can. That's because we have learned that our thoughts trigger our feelings, and our feelings fuel our behavior, and our behavior leads to our results.

For example, we have seen how replacing *Ought To* and *Have To* thinking with *Want To* thinking can help lead to more positive feelings and more positive results. We have learned that we cannot always choose the change in our lives, but we can always choose how we respond.

We have learned that feelings like guilt and anger are common but that we don't have to be slaves to those feelings. We have learned that asking for help is a sign of strength, not weakness. We have learned that there are others who want to help. By letting them help, we are allowing them to feel like they are making a difference—because they are.

We hope that all of this adds up to this realization too: Life can be tough, but you can be tougher. You have what you need inside. You have the internal fortitude and internal resources to see this thing through.

We hope also that you have realized you are not alone. There are millions of others all over the world going through very similar experiences in their roles as caregivers. There is an ever-expanding network of books and videos and websites and people to help you navigate this change in your life. We encourage you to tap into and contribute to that network as often as possible.

And finally, we hope you have come to realize that your path to happiness still exists. It may not be the path you once envisioned, and it may contain some unexpected and unwanted detours along the way, but the path is still there.

The path to happiness is lit with the light of hope and illuminated with the force of faith: faith in God, if you so choose; faith in yourself; faith in the basic goodness and decency of others.

Never stop seeking to travel that path. Because in the end, happiness and joy most often spring from life's stolen small moments rather than through big life events: the glimpse of a sunrise; the smell of cut grass; the sound of a child's laughter.

We encourage you to keep walking and pursuing that path of happiness and to walk it with others. Because we are all on this journey together. You are not alone. We appreciate you letting us join you as we walk that path together.

**Five Things to Do Now
to Pursue the Path of Happiness**

1. **Make a list of all the little things that bring you joy during the day.**

_____

_____

_____

_____

_____

_____

_____

_____

_____

_____

_____

_____

_____

_____

_____

_____

_____

_____

_____

_____

_____

_____

_____

_____

_____

_____

_____

2. **What are five things you are grateful for right now?**

_____

_____

_____

_____

_____

_____

3. **Sometimes the best way to help yourself is to help others.** Who do you know that could use an emotional boost or pick-me-up right about now? Write down their names and what you might do to offer them assistance, even if it just means picking up the phone to offer a word of encouragement.

_____

_____

_____

_____

---

4. **Sometimes laughter can be the best medicine.** Who or what are the things that make you laugh? Certain people you know? A favorite movie, book, or TV show? List them here, and make a commitment to reach out to that person or to watch that movie or show soon.

_____

_____

_____

_____

_____

_____

_____

_____

_____

_____

_____

_____

_____

5. **Put your mask on first.** Out of everything we have covered in this book, make a list of the top five things you can do to put your mask on first.

_____

_____

_____

_____

_____

_____

_____

_____

_____

_____

_____

_____

_____

_____

About The Authors

Scott Silknitter

Scott Silknitter is the founder of R.O.S. Therapy Systems. He designed and created the R.O.S. Play Therapy™ System, the *How Much Do You Know About* Series of themed activity books, the R.O.S. *BIG Book*, and the Engagement Program used by caregivers around the world. Starting with a simple backyard project to help his mother and father, Scott has dedicated his life to improving the quality of life for all seniors through meaningful education, entertainment, and activities. More information is available at www.ROSTherapySystems.com.

Gary Bradt

Dr. Gary Bradt is an author, clinical psychologist, leadership consultant, C-Suite executive coach, and speaker on the topic of adapting to and leading through change.

Dr. Bradt gained national attention in 2000 when Dr. Spencer Johnson, the renowned author of *Who Moved My Cheese? An Amazing Way to Deal with Change in Your Work and in Your Life* chose him as the leading speaker on the message of that blockbuster best-selling book which has sold over 35 million copies worldwide. *Cheese* gave thousands of people the chance to get acquainted with Gary's extraordinary ability to cut through their frustration and fear, and get to the heart of the matter; delivering powerful tools that help them adapt when going through change.

Dr. Bradt earned his BA in psychology from Duquesne University, in Pittsburgh PA. He earned his doctorate in clinical psychology from Hahnemann University and Hospital in Philadelphia, PA, which in 2007 honored him with the "Excellence in Professional Psychology" award. Only the second graduate to be so recognized at the time, this award underscored Dr. Bradt's contributions to the field of professional psychology through his achievements as an author, leadership consultant/coach, and world-class speaker. More information is available at www.garybradt.com.

1. Jonno Hanafin
   jonno@earthlink.net
   www.jonnohanafinassociates.com

Notes

Notes

Notes